# Yoga for Fools

2/22/19

for Susan Woodrow
with very best wishes,

[illegible signature]

# YOGA for Fools

Eric v.d. Luft

<< Gegensatz Press >>
2015

Cataloging in Publication:

Luft, Eric v.d. (Eric von der ), 1952- .
Yoga for fools / Eric v.d. Luft.
76 p. ; 22 cm.
ISBN 978-1-62130-747-1 (paperback)
ISBN 978-1-62130-745-7 (Kindle e-book)
ISBN 978-1-62130-744-0 (Smashwords e-book)
ISBN 978-1-62130-746-4 (Ingram e-book)
1. Yoga - Humor. I. Title.
RA 781.7 L83 2015 613.7 - dc22 AACR2
Library of Congress Control Number 2015944686



Distributed to the trade worldwide by:
Gegensatz Press
108 Deborah Lane
North Syracuse, NY 13212-1931
<www.gegensatzpress.com>

BISAC headings:
HEA025000 HEALTH & FITNESS / Yoga
HUM007000 HUMOR / Form / Parodies

Printed on acid-free paper. ∞

## Disclaimer!

What appears on the even-numbered, left-side pages is genuine information about yoga; but what appears on the odd-numbered, right-side pages is parody. Please don't mix them up! Neither the author, the publisher, nor even Lord Krishna himself, will assume any responsibility for any consequences if you do.

While yoga is essentially an ascetic discipline, and requires no specific adherence to Hinduism or any other religion, it is nevertheless true that yoga developed out of pre-Vedic, Vedic, and Vedantic Hinduism, and has been around in some form for about 3000 years. The Hindu god who is mostly closely identified with yoga is Shiva, the god of destruction. That is no mere coincidence.

It is thus probably best to treat yoga as a secular activity.

Never mind that this disclaimer appears on an odd-numbered, right-side page.

# Pranayama

Yoga is a bunch of poses (asanas) wrapped around the breath. Breathing is yoga's most important aspect and requires the most discipline. The purpose of the asanas is to help you breathe - and thus to help you live longer, healthier, and happier - by opening the joints; stretching the muscles, tendons, and ligaments; and generally loosening the body and expanding its possibilities.

The most basic breathing technique is ujjayi. Here's how to do it: Shut your mouth. Relax. Breathe only through the nose. Shove the belly out, thus lowering the diaphragm and making more room for the lungs to expand, then inhale slowly and deliberately into, first the lower chest, then the middle chest, and finally the upper chest all the way up to the larynx. When your whole torso is completely full of air, begin to exhale, legato, lentissimo, finally sucking the navel into the spine to squeeze out the last little bit of air. With each new breath, gradually increase the total volume of air exchanged until you are breathing only a few times per minute.

Slow it down. Control it. Control yourself. Yoga is all about control. The word "yoga" means "joining" and refers to the natural union between yourself and the universe. Making that union harmonious requires a ton of control on your part. The art of controlling the breath is called pranayama.

On the other hand, maybe you don't enjoy breathing. Maybe you would prefer not to.

There are several ways to indulge your masochism and ensure your misery in this regard.

Try holding your breath as you do the asanas. Tense up. Feel your body shake. Concentrate on not breathing. Consider that the pose is everything and the breath is nothing. Focus on the tightness in your lungs as it radiates throughout your entire being. Be competitive. Defy the universe. Notice how your limbs soon tire, how your forehead sweats even in a cool room, and how your equilibrium disappears.

Stand under a sign that says "Positively No Smoking!" light up a butt, suck off a big drag, and proclaim loudly to the world, "Negatively Some Smoking!"

Get a job in a coal mine, a gypsum factory, a dusty warehouse, a toxic chemical environment, or any other oxygen-challenged venue, and don't wear a mask or any other kind of respiratory protection.

Grow a set of gills and become aquatic. Lurk in a lagoon and become anaerobic. Write if it works.

## Alternate Nostril Breathing (Nadi Shodhana)

One major goal of yoga is to get your chakras all lined up and working for you in an orderly way. Proper breathing does that. Chakras are dedicated energy hubs arranged vertically from the top of your head to your anus. They are the colors of the rainbow (Roy G. Biv) and each has its own special sound (bija mantra). The mantra "Om" is shared by the top two chakras. Philologically, "Om" is related to the Latin "omnis," which means "all." From top to bottom, your chakras are:

1. Crown chakra (Sahasrara) - violet - Om
2. Third eye chakra (Ajna) - indigo - Om
3. Throat chakra (Vishuddha) - blue - Ham
4. Heart center chakra (Anahata) - green - Yam
5. Umbilical chakra (Manipura) - yellow - Ram
6. Genital chakra (Svadhishthana) - orange - Vam
7. Root chakra (Muladhara) - red - Lam

To cleanse your whole system, body, mind, and spirit, put the tip of your middle finger on - not in - your third eye. That's your pivot point. Close one nostril with your thumb. Exhale. Inhale. Open that nostril and close the other with your pinky. Exhale. Inhale. Pivot again. Repeat. Real yogis can do nadi shodhana without using their fingers, which in this case are like training wheels on a bicycle.

## Alternate Orifice Breathing (Buti Snuti)

Topologically, a human being is a donut (or perhaps, if born between late April and late May, a torus). This means that there is a single hole that goes all the way through the body. It's a very long hole with lots of twists and turns, but it's still only one hole. There's a threefold opening of the hole at one end and a onefold opening at the other end.

We typically breathe through either the nostrils or the mouth or both (the three openings of the hole at the front end). But there's no good reason why we couldn't breathe through the opening of the hole at the other end instead. All that this change would require is a bit of self-control. Remember that yoga is all about control. Mind over matter. Spirit over flesh. Unity over diversity. Resolution! Just do it!

To achieve buti snuti, close your mouth, hold your nose, and try to breathe. Can't do it? Well, maybe that's because you didn't empty your stomach and bowels first. Unless you cleanse everything south of the esophagus, alternate orifice breathing is awfully difficult - if not impossible - with all that glop in the way. So, grab a nice long book, have a seat in the bathroom, and don't eat or drink anything for three days. Or, if you're in a hurry, you could use one of those colonoscopy preps that works overnight.

## Root Lock (Mula Bandha)

A bandha is a connection, a bond, an impediment, a restraint, a dam, or a lock. In yoga there are three fundamental bandhas: the throat lock (jalandhara bandha), the stomach lock (uddiyana bandha), and the root lock (mula bandha). Maha bandha, the "great bandha" or the "big lock," is the simultaneous performance of all three.

Like a dam on a river, a bandha stops the regular flow but at the same time creates a reservoir of energy (prana) by concentrating it around and in a certain chakra. By dropping the chin to the chest while at the same time lifting it upward, you close both the trachea and esophagus temporarily and stimulate the vishuddha. By exhaling the diaphragm up into the chest as far as it will go and sucking the abdominal viscera as far back toward the spine as they will go, you tone the abdomen and stimulate the manipura.

But by far the most powerful and most interesting of the three bandhas is the root lock. It's like a unisex Kegel maneuver. Exhale, then use all your perineal muscles to squish your anus shut tight and to pull it up into your abdomen, while keeping the spine straight. This, if held indefinitely, will really lock you up.

## Root Unlock (Mula Flatulentha)

The root lock is difficult to maintain, especially for those who follow a vegetarian diet and even more especially for those who eat a lot of beans. But we don't fight against nature. We go with the flow. We accept the realities of the lower tract and learn to work with them.

So, relax.

Really relax.

If you've ever been to an Indian restaurant, you know that this cuisine features all sorts of liquidy concoctions like raita, chutneys, curries, kheer, etc., and that its main dishes are soupy and contain hardly any meat, except for an occasional chicken, lamb, or goat dish, and are more like lumpy sauces on top of rice than real entrees. Most of the food is fragrant or spicy or both. Having a steady diet of this stuff makes the root unlock almost automatic.

Thus we achieve the "sacred sound" which Dante describes in the *Divine Comedy*, *Inferno*, canto XXI, line 139: "ed agli avea del cul fatto trompetta." "Om" is the sacred sound of the universe as a whole, but what we are creating here is the sacred sound of the other end of the universe as a hole.

## Mountain (Tadasana)

This is the basic position of standing strength. It looks effortless and simple, but it is really quite a vigorous and complicated asana.

Be perfectly vertical, as if there were an invisible string pulling you straight up through the crown of your head. Build your mountain, i.e., build yourself into a mountain, from the ground up. Root all four corners of each foot solidly into the ground. Engage your legs. Contract your calves. Lift your patellas. Tighten your quads. Compress your buttocks. Tuck your tailbone in. Suck your tummy in. Expand your chest. Lengthen your neck. Breathe deeply and slowly. Get taller, straighter, and harder with every breath. Roll your shoulders up and back, then let your arms hang soft and limp. Your whole body should be perfectly centered and balanced.

## Upward Salute (Urdhva Hastasana)

From tadasana, stick your arms straight out to each side, palms up, horizontally, at right angles to your body, as far as they will reach. Inhale your palms together directly over your head, as high as they will reach. With each exhale, stabilize. With each inhale, lengthen your whole body, making it as tall as possible, but keeping both feet flat on the floor.

## Strip-Mined Mountain (Appalachiasana)

Standing in tadasana for any amount of time takes quite a bit of effort. You might think that mountains have it easy, just sitting around for millions of years with pine trees growing on them, bears rambling all over them, and rivers flowing off them; but in fact mountains have it tough. Wind erosion, water erosion, ice erosion ... and worst of all, strip miners who lop the tops right off them just to get their mitts on a few lumps of coal.

So, to honor these long-suffering mounds of earth and rock, we will crumble into dust. But don't just stand in tadasana until you crumble; be proactive instead, start the crumbling process yourself. Drop your head onto your chest. Let your knees buckle. Get wobbly. Fall down. Remember those pratfalls you learned how to do in junior high dramatics club? Well, that's useful knowledge now, isn't it?

## Abandoned Shack (Kondemdasana)

From urdhva hastasana, gradually let your entire body go limp from the top down. Exhale completely. Soften all your muscles. Release all your tension. Relax all your joints. Slowly collapse into nothing. Fade into the earth. Become one with that which is and that which is not.

## Child (Balasana)

You need a rest.

Kneel with your insteps on the floor and about hip distance apart. Sit on your heels. Bend forward and bring your chest down onto the top of your thighs. Gently place your forehead on the floor as far in front of you as it will go. Keep your butt down as low as you can. Stretch your arms out in front of you as far as you can. Feel it in the back of your shoulders.

From balasana, you can easily flow into cobra (page 42 below) - and back again - and again.

## Thread the Needle (Parsva Balasana)

From balasana, stick your right arm straight up in the air, sweep it under your left armpit, twist your upper body to the left, and put your right cheek on the floor, all while keeping your left arm stretched forward. Return to balasana and do it on the other side.

## Rabbit (Sasangasana)

From balasana, bring your forehead back to touch the front of your lower thighs between your knees, reach back and grab your heels, and stick your butt up in the air as high as you can. This creates a good stretch for your spine.

## Naughty Child (Bratasana)

Go to the nearest dark corner of the room, or, if outside, to the nearest windowless wall. Without touching this structure, but being as close to it as possible, face it directly, gaze straight ahead, and go into tadasana (page 12 above).

Stand perfectly still. Make no sound. Breathe normally. Do not mutter under your breath. Do not curse. You may, if you wish, hold your breath until you turn blue.

Meditate on the pure magnificence, omnipotence, omniscience, omnibenevolence, and mercy of your parents. Acknowledge how unworthy you are to be their child. In this way, you will regain your self-esteem as you gradually become aware of how lucky and privileged you are to be allowed to bask in their unconditional love.

Remain in this pose until you have calmed down, realized the error of your ways, learned not to blame anyone else for your mistakes, and achieved cosmic serenity. At this point you may turn around, exhale, bow your head, and meekly step forward while chanting a sincere and contrite "I'm sorry" as your context-specific mantra. Cheerfully ask forgiveness and smile gratefully when you receive it.

## Hero (Virasana)

Kneel with your insteps on the floor and your legs together. Sit on your heels. Sit up very straight. Remember that invisible string pulling you up through the crown of your head. Roll your shoulders back and down, straighten your arms, and place your palms on top of your knees. Your hips, shoulders, and ears should all be in a line perpendicular to the floor. Be bold. Be strong. Be tall. Be resolute.

Virasana has plenty of variants, for example:

1. To invigorate your shoulders, arms, and hands, make cactus arms. Hold both arms straight out to your sides with both forearms straight up at a 90-degree angle to the upper arms. Spread the fingers wide. Pivot the palms inward and outward.

2. To get a deeper stretch into the knees, keep your knees together but spread your ankles far enough apart so that you can sit on the floor.

3. To torment yourself and ruin your knees, from variant 2, grab each elbow over your head, tuck your tailbone in, and carefully lean straight back all the way to the floor, slowly inhaling, slowly exhaling, and keeping your spine long.

## Coward (Wimpasana)

Be afraid. Wince at the slightest irregularity, oddity, disturbance, or unexpected appearance. Go into balasana (page 14 above), preferably under or behind a large, solid, stable object, if you can find one. If you can't find one, be even more afraid.

From balasana, become very, very small. Shut your eyes. Pull your face down toward your chest. Stack your forearms over the back of your head, one palm pressing on the nape of your neck, the other pressing on the back of that hand. Your mantra is now a whimper, a sniffle, or a whine. Express this mantra freely, but be very bashful about it, quiet, almost silent. You don't want anyone or anything else to know that you are there or that you even exist. In fact, you just barely exist. Meditate on the truth of Shakespeare's *Julius Caesar*, II, ii, 37-40: "Of all the wonders that I yet have heard, • It seems to me most strange that men should fear; • Seeing that death, a necessary end, • Will come when it will come."

Try very hard *not* to go into a spontaneous root unlock (page 11 above) - although it may seem impossible to avoid - but instead work to maintain a firm root lock. Tense up. Tremble. Shiver. Shudder. Fail. Accept defeat. Feel worthless.

## Cat-Cow (Marjariasana-Bitilasana)

Get on your hands and knees, with your wrists right under your shoulders, your knees right under your hips, insteps on the floor, and fingers spread out. Hands should be shoulder width apart and knees should be hip width apart. Arms and thighs should be vertical. Your back should be horizontal and level. This is called table (bharmanasana) - but more about that below on page 54. Relax. Breathe.

Exhale fully, pushing your belly button into your spine, emptying your lungs, dropping your head, and arching your back upward. This is the cat phase (marjariasana). You can meow if you want. Or purr. Or hiss.

Inhale fully, pushing your whole belly out, filling your lungs, raising your head, and arching your back downward. This is the cow phase (bitilasana). Moo if it mooves you.

Alternate cat and cow slowly and deliberately. Exhale into cat. Inhale into cow.

This is a wonderful pair of complementary asanas to work your abs, develop flexibility in your spine, increase chest and lung capacity, provide aerobic cardiovascular exercise, and reduce your phlegm.

## Politician (Scumbaggasana)

While in cow, open your mouth and tell a lie. Even better, open your mouth on just one side, but tell the lie out of the other side. This requires practice. Law school helps.

As you exhale into cat, keep going. That is, don't stop at the usual upward arched position. Continue smoothly, moving your head toward your root chakra. This might be difficult for ordinary people, but not for real politicians, because they have no backbone. Keep trying. If you ever want to get elected, you'll have to master this. Open up the spaces between those vertebrae.

Eventually your sahasrara will touch your muladhara. Keep pushing. Go as far as you can. Then inhale again into cow. Tell another lie. You will find that your recent contact with your root chakra has enhanced your ability to tell bolder, more convincing, more creative, more exotic, more knavish, and more absurd lies. Keep alternating.

Any middling politician can insert the crown chakra into the root chakra. A more accomplished politician can get the ajna in there. But only a consummate politician can insert the whole head into the muladhara all the way to the vishuddha.

## Tree (Vrksasana)

From tadasana (page 12 above), find your drishti. A drishti is a stationary point of focus that enables you to concentrate fully, without thinking, without trying, without distractions. Your drishti is very personal and belongs to no one but you. It might be an imaginary point a few inches in front of your (crossed) eyes; it might be a spot on the wall; it might be your guru's ass; it might be anything at all.

Once you have found and fixed your drishti and erased all content from your mind, shift your weight slightly to one side, anchor all four corners of your foot, especially the pinky toe, on that side, then lift your other foot off the floor. Balance! You can rest your heel in your crotch or, if you prefer, your sole on your instep, your toes on your thigh. Take your pick. Rest your foot on anything you want, except the inside of your knee. You could even kick your leg out and grab your big toe in a lock (utthita hasta padangusthasana; page 48 below).

Stand still. Breathe. Move your arms or your raised foot if you want, but do it deliberately. Try a little backbend. Or maybe a sidebend. Be a saguaro with cactus arms (page 16 above) or a mighty oak against the wind. If you stagger, stumble, wiggle, waver, tremble, or fall over, then you've done it wrong.

## Fallen Tree (Timberasana)

Failing at vrksasana does not mean that you have failed as a person, or even as a yogi.

Use this minor disappointment to your spiritual advantage. Don't wallow in so much self-pity that you turn into a miserable schmuck. Use your innate power and gumption to lift you out of this transient muddle and make us all proud of you.

From your crumpled position on the floor, assess yourself. No broken limbs? No damage to your trunk? No dry rot? No termites? You're fine.

Believe that you're fine! Start your new growth! Re-establish your roots. Build yourself. Nourish yourself. Have a drink of water. Cover your feet with mulch. Arise!

Get back into tadasana. Find your drishti again. Anchor that left foot. Lift up that right foot. Kick it out! Reach for the sky. Be solid! Be tough! You're a stalwart, deep-rooted hickory that nothing can either bend or break, not a feeble, shallow-rooted willow at the mercy of the weather. You're a stately, majestic redwood, not a pathetic, misshapen scrub pine. Watch out for lumberjacks - but otherwise, don't even think about it. Channel Joyce Kilmer!

## Bridge (Setubandhasana)

Relax supine on the floor with your arms straight alongside your body, palms down. Inhale your feet toward your body until your heels are up against your butt. Keep your feet flat and knees together. Exhale. Push your palms firmly down into the floor. Inhale and gradually roll your backbone up off the floor from the coccyx to the base of the skull - or as far as you can comfortably go - one vertebra at a time. Roll it up! Imagine that you're the famous aerial bridge in Duluth, Minnesota, slowly rising to allow a ship to pass beneath you. Now roll it back down, one vertebra at a time.

## Staff (Dandasana)

Sit up straight with your legs together and sticking straight out in front of you. Roll your shoulders back, straighten your arms, and put your palms next to your butt on the floor, with the fingers together and pointing straight ahead. Flex your feet and point your toes toward your head. Your body should form a perfect 90-degree angle: legs horizontal; torso, arms, neck, and head vertical. Again remember that invisible string pulling you up through the crown of your head. With each inhale, push the legs farther out and the head higher up. With each exhale, push the butt farther down and farther back.

## Tunnel (Undhawattasana)

This asana assists alternate orifice breathing (page 9 above). Recall that the body is a natural donut. We will now elongate and streamline that donut.

Lie down, either prone, supine, or on your side. It doesn't matter. Whichever is most comfortable for you. Breathe. Concentrate. Become aware of each internal organ. Focus in particular on your entire alimentary canal - the hole of the donut. Unkink, uncoil, widen, shorten, and align your esophagus, duodenum, and especially your intestines. This requires extreme internal control, but if done correctly, it will reduce resistance all along the channel between both openings of the donut hole.

Note the resemblance of the sacred mantra "Om" to "Ohm," the measure of resistance. Ebb and flow. In and out. The more Oms, the fewer Ohms.

You may, if you wish, erect a toll booth at each end.

## Wet Noodle (Limpasana)

Loosen everything up. Slack it off. Wilt. Droop. Let it all dangle. Embrace your softness. Become one with your essential flaccidity. Take it easy. No rules. No directions. Just get comfortable.

## Spinal Twist or "Half Fish" (Ardha Matsyendrasana)

From dandasana (page 22 above), bend your right knee and put your right sole on the floor with the outside of the right foot touching the left thigh and the right heel as close to your left hip as it will go. Again remember the invisible string. Push your butt down and pull your head up. Put the outside of the left elbow against the outside of the right knee and bend the left forearm straight up. Stick your right arm straight out horizontally to the right and gaze at the tip of its middle finger. Sweep that arm around back to the right, keeping that gaze fixed. Put your right palm on the floor with the heel of that hand against your left butt cheek. Stare over your right shoulder as far as your neck will go. Return to dandasana and do the twist on the other side.

## Sage Twist (Marichyasana)

Same as above, but clasp hands behind your back.

## Alligator Twist (Jathara Parivartanasana)

Lie supine with your arms stretched straight out at right angles to your body, palms pressing down hard. Keep your legs together, lift them up as high as possible with knees bent or not, bring them far over to the left, and turn your head to the right. Now switch: legs to the right and head to the left. Repeat like windshield wipers.

### Dying Gaul (Museicapitoliniasana)

From any position, drop down on your butt and catch yourself with your straight right arm from falling all the way. Bend forward, trying to sit up. Your left leg is sticking out to the left, with the knee bent and the sole flat on the ground. Your right leg is bent under your left, with the inside of the right foot just below, but not touching, the left thigh, and the outside of this foot is on the ground. Your left hand is resting softly just above your right knee. Soften your neck and put your chin on your right collarbone. Breathe desperately, with less and less power - diminuendo - as you watch your life ebb away through the wound in your right breast.

### Oliver Twist (Artfuldodgasana)

Starve for three months, subsisting on gruel, then gather up all your remaining strength, compose yourself, stand tall, stride forward, and boldly speak your mantra, "Please, Sir, I want some more."

### Peppermint Twist (Jhohi Di Nicolasana)

Inhale. Go around. Exhale. And around. Inhale. Go up. Exhale. Come down. Inhale. Count to three. Exhale. Kick. Inhale. Count to three. Exhale. Jump. Inhale. Sing your song. Exhale. Don't take long.

## Dancer (Natarajasana)

From tadasana, bend your right knee so that your heel is as close as possible to your right butt cheek, then grab your right ankle with your right hand. Inhale your left arm straight up, palm forward, fingers together, trying to touch the sky. Find your drishti. Stay steady while slowly, slowly bending forward from the waist, keeping your left leg and both arms straight, and your left arm near your ear and in line with your spine. Your right heel will naturally move away from your butt. Stop bending forward when your right thigh and your left arm both become parallel to the floor. Your left palm should be downward. Your right arm might bend.

Well, you can't really dance in this position, but it's a silhouette artist's dream. Don't forget to breathe.

You still want to dance, right? Then let's boogie! Experiment a little!

Try the yoga toe lock (page 48 below) on your big right toe and wiggle your right leg around. Put your right sole on the back of your head.

Bend your right elbow and wave it up and down.

Then try the whole thing from the other side.

### Singer (Mikjaggasana)

Proceed through your entire repertoire of standing asanas. Keep moving! Strut! Tease! Pose! Act like God! Make sure that everyone sees, knows, and feels just how gorgeous and wonderful you are. But remember, the difference between God and a rock star is that God doesn't prance around pretending to be a rock star.

### Manager (Tomparkerasana)

Sit in sukhasana (page 34 below) and order the singer around. Don't forget to manipulate.

### Choreographer (Balanchinasana)

Sit in sukhasana and order the dancer around. Don't forget to look smug and disgusted.

### Producer (Diddlerasana)

Sit in sukhasana and order the engineer around. Don't forget to diddle with the knobs.

### Impresario (Bilgrammasana)

Sit in sukhasana and order everyone around. Don't forget to count your money.

## Extended Triangle (Utthita Trikonasana)

From tadasana, stay strong and spread your legs wide apart so that the floor and the inside of each leg form an equilateral triangle. Balance. Focus. Be tall. Keep your knees straight. Inhale your right arm straight up, palm inward, fingers together, reaching for the sky. Turn your left foot out 90 degrees. Lunge left so that your left arm and left shin are touching, parallel, and vertical; and your right arm, torso, and right leg are all in line. Now do it on the other side.

## Revolving Triangle (Parivrtta Trikonasana)

Alternately, instead of reaching one arm up, reach both arms horizontally, palms downward, parallel to the floor. Turn your left foot out 90 degrees. Bend sideways to the left, sharply from the waist so that your left palm touches the outside of your left ankle, your arms are vertical, and your right hand reaches for the sky. Turn your torso 180 degrees so that your right palm is touching the inside of your left ankle, your arms are vertical, and your left hand reaches for the sky.

Return to standing upright with arms extended horizontally. Do the foot turn, sideways bend, ankle touch, sky reach, and torso turn to the right this time. Repeat until you get dizzy.

## Möbius Strip (Mauritsescherasana)

Lie on your right side at full length. Straighten your body, point your toes, and stretch your fingertips over your head as far from your toes as possible, as in urdhva hastasana. Breathe slowly and smoothly. With each inhale, do a little backbend, each one a little farther than the last one. With each exhale, stabilize. Eventually the letter "C" that you are forming with your body as your legs and arms go behind you and your belly sticks out will become the letter "O." When it does, grab your left (top) foot with your left (top) hand, your right (bottom) foot with your right (bottom) hand, and hold on.

Continue to breathe steadily and calmly. With each inhale, rotate the top half of your body, above the waist, a bit to the right, each increment a little farther than the last one. You are proceeding toward a half-twist of your spine. To complete the half-twist, grab your left (top) foot with your right (top) hand, your right (bottom) foot with your left (top) hand, and hold on. If you've done it right, then an ant crawling down your body from the back of your head should end up on your face.

Now do it from the other side, with everything reversed. Being either an invertebrate or a cartoon character helps.

## Eagle (Garudasana)

From tadasana, bring your arms in front of you with your elbows bent upward and your left elbow in the crook of your right. Keep your hands straight up, don't bend your wrists, and twist your forearms around so that the palmsides of the fingers of the right hand are resting on the palm of your left hand. Everything from your elbows to your fingertips should be straight in a vertical line.

Bend your left knee and balance on your left foot. Cross your right thigh over your left, bend your right knee, and hook your right instep behind your left calf. Bend your knees to squat down even lower, and at the same time raise your hands skyward until you feel like your shoulders might dislocate.

Now return to tadasana and try it the other way, with the right arm inside the left and the left leg over the right.

Believe it or not, this asana tones your calves, ankles, and shoulders.

It's a bit hard to imagine how an eagle could fly in this position, but apparently the ancient gurus who named these asanas exercised some poetic license.

## Rainbow Lorikeet (Pollachromatasana)

Your yoga mat is your private island. You can do whatever you want on your mat and no one will judge you. What happens on your mat stays on your mat.

The ultimate yoga mat would resemble the mat of the 1966 Milton Bradley game, Twister®, which had four rows of big colored circles, six green, six yellow, six blue, and six red: twenty-four circles altogether. This game was a godsend for horny but sexually frustrated teenagers. Up to six people could play, and a seventh would be the spinner, whose job was to spin a dial to tell the contestants where to put the left foot, right foot, left hand, and right hand.

So, here we go!

Left foot on green.
Right foot on red.
Left hand on blue,
Right hand on yellow.
Left foot on red.
Right foot on green.
Left hand on green.
Right hand on red.

Breathe! Balance! Don't fall over!

## Boat (Navasana)

From dandasana (page 22 above), bend the knees and grab the back of each thigh just behind the knee. Inhale. Lean back, keeping the spine straight and long. Lift your feet off the floor and straighten your legs. Let go of your thighs but keep your hands next to the outside of your knees, fingers together, hands sticking straight out away from your shoulders.

The line from the top of your head, sahasrara, to your butt, muladhara, should now be at a 45-degree angle to the floor. Similarly, the line from your heels to your butt should also be at a 45-degree angle to the floor. Your arms should be straight, level, and horizontal.

You are now a boat. You do not want to be leaky. You want to be taut and shipshape. Performing the root lock prevents leaks.

You are not a racing skiff, a clipper, a dreadnought, or a dhow. You are more like a coracle or a tiny papyrus canoe. You must stay upright to stay afloat. You have no keel. Stability is a problem. Balancing on your butt isn't easy.

Roll with the waves and don't let barnacles grow on your hull.

## Shipwreck (Davyjonesasana)

From navasana, perform the root unlock and let the leaking begin. Yo ho ho!

Become unstable. Feel like you're breaking up. Capsize! Fall roughly to one side or the other. Women and children first!

Go down once. Bob back up. Try to breathe.

Go down twice. Bob back up. Sputter.

Go down three times. Glub glub!

Sink! The captain goes down with the ship, settling on the ocean floor, sleeping with the fishes.

Remember "Loosen Up" by the Nazz of Philadelphia (1971), done in response to "Tighten Up" by Archie Bell and the Drells of Houston, Texas (1968)? Well, this is the nautical equivalaent. So loosen up on the hull and grease on a tuna fish hoagie. For an extra kick, use a live tuna.

## Bermuda Triangle (Paranorma Trikonasana)

Same as above, but instead of sinking, just vanish into thin air.

## Easy Sitting (Sukhasana)

This is the basic cross-legged position, familiar to us all since we were kids. But do you really believe that yoga would let us off so easy? Not a chance!

## Half Lotus (Siddhasana)

From dandasana (page 22 above), bring the sole of one foot to the inside of the opposite thigh. Then put the outside of the other foot into the angle of the opposite knee.

## Full Lotus (Padmasana)

From dandasana, bring the instep of the left foot to rest in the angle between the right lower abdomen and the top of the right thigh. Then bring the instep of the right foot over the left leg to rest in the angle between the left lower abdomen and the top of the left thigh. Or do the right foot first and the left foot second. It doesn't matter. Sit up straight with your hands resting comfortably on your knees. Breathe.

A lotus is a gorgeous flower with a huge cup-shaped symmetrical bloom and umpteen bladelike petals. Its circularity is a symbol of universality and perfection. Its petals symbolize the unity of the many in the one. We wish to achieve serenity when we are sitting calmly cross-legged like this, but not necessarily to resemble the actual flower.

## Lotus Seven Series Two (Karwuntwentiseeasana)

In dandasana (page 22 above), breathe normally but deeply and intensely. Narrow your eyes to slits, look straight ahead with strong purpose, but keep your peripheral vision as wide as possible. Stay aware of everything within you and around you. Cultivate a self-satisfied smirk.

Stand up. Stride decisively forward. Look straight ahead with a piercing, penetrating gaze. Lose your peripheral vision. Tunnel vision is now appropriate only because you are now in a tunnel.

Stomp back and forth. Be fierce. Pound things. Yell. Resign.

Turn around 180 degrees. Go back into dandasana. Engage everything. Believe that you have won. Become unaware of what is happening behind you.

Slow down. Recover your normal, deep, intense breathing, your peripheral vision, and especially your self-satisfied smirk. Begin to have trouble breathing. Spontaneously fall back into savasana (page 74 below) and remain in this position until you lose track of time, place, space, and motion.

Wake up in the Village.

### High Lunge (Alanasana)

From downward dog (page 40 below), inhale and step one foot quickly between your hands so that all three point forward in line and your arms and that calf are perpendicular to the floor. Exhale and gather your wits. Inhale your arms straight up, as in virabhadrasana I (page 68 below), do a backbend, and gaze either straight ahead or slightly upward.

### Low Lunge (Anjaneyasana)

From downward dog, step one foot forward as in the high lunge, but, instead of keeping the other leg straight, put the other knee, shin, and instep all on the floor. Place one palm on your front knee, your other palm on the back of that hand, inhale, and use your arms to push into a backbend. Push hard!

### Runner's Lunge (Ardha Hanumanasana)

From tadasana, bend forward sharply and put your palms on the floor, fingers together and forward, just outside your feet. Inhale. Step one foot back as far as you can, landing on your toes and keeping that leg straight. Your other leg should now be at a 90-degree angle, foot flat on the floor, shin vertical, thigh horizontal and parallel to the floor. Push your chest and head forward and gaze straight ahead.

## Thrust (Coupasana)

With one hand behind your back, step in and out of various lunges. Wave the other hand wildly back and forth. Dance! Keep your balance. Watch out for the other yogis' parries (see below). Don't fall over or you're done for.

## Parry (Voltasana)

With one hand behind your back, step in and out of various lunges. Wave the other hand wildly from side to side and around in circles. Dance! Jump! Feint! Keep your balance. Use your reflexes. Watch out for the other yogis' thrusts (see above). Don't fall over or you're done for.

## Runner's Mark (Getsetgoasana)

From tadasana (page 12 above), step one foot back slightly, bend your knees, and crouch down so that your weight is on the balls of your feet. With your thumbs and index fingers on the floor just behind an imaginary line perpendicular to your body, turn both hands outward from the wrists so that all eight fingers are parallel, the four fingertips on each hand point 180 degrees away from the four on the other hand, and the two thumb tips point toward each other. Lean into it, keep your head up, and fix your gaze on your intention, straight ahead. Tense up, ready to spring forward.

## Lion (Simhasana)

In virasana (page 16 above), make funny faces and stretch out your arms like a lion's claws. Is that all there is to it? Not quite.

Straighten your arms, tense them up, and push your palms down hard on your knees. Inhale. Puff your chest out and sit tall. Open your eyes and mouth as wide as possible - and even wider. Spread your fingers and thumbs as far apart as they will go - and even farther - painfully far. Stick your tongue out as far as you can, bend it down and try to touch the tip of your chin with the tip of your tongue. Be tense all over. Hold your breath in this position for as long as you can. Then exhale, soften, and relax.

Repeat. Again. As often as you want.

Simhasana exercises your chin, wrists, neck, hands, and jaw. It deeply tones facial skin, prevents sags, and removes wrinkles. Some say that it stimulates the salivary glands, larynx, throat, capillaries, and thyroid, thus improving digestion, strengthening the voice, making breathing and swallowing easier, enhancing circulation, and fostering general well being. This is probably true. Others say that it gives you sex appeal, builds your equity, and helps your chances of winning the lottery. This is not true.

## Warthog (Afro Piggasana)

Be tough, stout, and adaptable. Look sallow, ugly, and menacing. Trot around aimlessly on all fours. Don't worry about your appearance. Vanity has no place in your life. Stick your lower teeth out over your upper lip. Be proud of the bumps all over your face. Be at home with yourself and satisfied with what you are. For you, life is not a problem.

If you're a boar and you see a sow and another boar, fight him over her. If you're a sow, find two boars to fight over you.

If you see a bug, eat it. If you see a plant, eat it. Eat whatever you please. If you think there's a tasty root underground, crouch down and dig it up with your chin. That's right. With the tusks on your chin.

If you're a sow, get together with other sows, grunt, snort, howl, chirp, snuggle, banter, and pick the bugs off each other. Wow! What a busy social life!

If you're a boar, just go off by yourself, strut your stuff, mark your territory with your own special scent, and threaten the other boars. Such fun!

The benefits of this asana are difficult to pin down. There probably aren't any.

## Downward Dog (Adho Mukha Svanasana)

This is a feline to canine transformation. From marjariasana (page 18 above) - or a lunge, balasana (page 14 above), or some other low, downward-facing asana - straighten your legs and line up your arms, head, and torso. Lead with your butt. End up on your palms and toes with your butt way up in the air. Your body should now form an equilateral triangle, with one side the floor from your hands to your feet, one side from your hands to your butt, and one side from your butt to your feet.

Relax your head and neck. You can shake your head gently back and forth if you want, but keep your neck and spine in line and don't let your head droop.

Pedal your feet up and down on your toes. Or bounce your heels up and down in unison. Be happy. Wag your tail.

## Butterfly (Baddha Konasana)

From dandasana (page 22 above), bring both heels into your crotch and bring both soles together so that your knees are sticking straight out to the sides. Clasp your hands around your toes and sit up tall. If you wish, you can flap your legs up and down like a butterfly.

### Hydrant Dog (Mutpisasana)

From adho mukha svanasana, grin and raise one leg high and sideways. Put that leg down, waddle on all fours a few steps, sniff the floor where you just raised your leg, waddle a few more steps, then grin and raise your other leg high and sideways. Repeat as many times as you wish.

### Variant: Tree Dog (Vrksamutpisasana)

Perform the same motions as above, but raise your leg at someone who is doing vrksasana.

### Mosquito (Malariasana)

The tree dog may annoy your guru and the other yogis, but it will never annoy them nearly as much as the mosquito. If you are inclined toward being very annoying, this is just the asana for you.

Buzz all around the yoga studio, keeping out of sight and out of reach of the other yogis, but fly up into their faces when they least expect it, then fly out of reach again before they can slap you. This will hone your reflexes and your evasive skills.

If one of them ever succeeds in slapping you, you must instantly go into savasana (page 74 below).

### Crocodile (Makarasana)

There are many prone asanas, some easy, some very difficult. This is the easiest, so we'll start with it.

Lie prone, legs together, insteps on the floor. Fold your arms in front of you and rest your forehead on them. Melt into the floor. Lurk there. That's it.

### Sphinx (Salamba Bhujangasana)

Lie prone, legs together, insteps on the floor, palms and forearms pointing forward, flat on the floor, elbows directly under your shoulders, upper arms vertical, and head up, looking straight ahead. You are now naturally in the sphinx position, whether you like it or not.

### Cobra (Bhujangasana)

As you lie prone with legs together, put your palms flat on the floor, directly under your shoulders, with fingers together, arms and elbows as close to your body as possible, and hands pointing forward. Relax your shoulders, inhale, and slowly push your chest up as far as it will go, while keeping your thighs in full contact with the floor. Bend your spine, neck, and head back, but don't throw them back. Exhale and return to prone. Repeat.

## Mongoose (Rikki Tikki Tavasana)

The mongoose is the nemesis of the cobra. As an Indian gray mongoose, you would very much enjoy killing cobras and going totally berserk while doing it. Become one with your mongoose body (herpestes sharira).

Lurk in some convenient and comfortable pose, such as balasana (page 14 above) or marjariasana-bitilasana (page 18 above) , waiting for your guru or one of your fellow yogis to go into bhujangasana, then leap up! Dance merrily on your toes all around your cobra. Be agile. Taunt. Bait. Make eye contact if possible. Hold off. Stretch out. Intimidate. Skulk. Evade. Tease. Scrutinize. Conserve your energy. Anticipate getting around in back for a mighty jump to deliver that one final devastating bite to the back of the head. Don't let your cobra bite you.

## Sidewinder (Boogalooasana)

Lie prone and perform ardha chandrasana (page 52 below). Now do it on the other side. Again! Double time! Bring your arms down to your sides, loosen up, move your shoulders up and down, keep shimmying from side to side, let your neck, knees, and waist go all rubbery, and do the horizontal boogaloo. How fast can you go?

### Upward Dog (Urdhva Mukha Svanasana)

Similar to cobra (page 42 above), but more intense. Instead of your palms, thighs, knees, and insteps touching the floor, now it's only palms and insteps.

### Plank (Chaturanga Dandasana)

This is sort of like the old-fashioned push-up that you did in gym class. But not entirely. It's a just a bit tougher and more complicated. The trick is to stay absolutely flat from the heels to the back of the head. Move gradually from cobra (page 42 above) through upward dog into plank. Or move gradually from downward dog (page 40 above) into plank.

### Gate (Parighasana)

From virasana (page 16 above), stick your right leg straight out to the side, knee unbent, foot extended, sole on the floor - if you can manage it, or if you can't, then the heel, not the inside of the foot, on the floor. Inhale both arms straight out, Exhale, Inhale your left arm up over toward the right while your right arm slides down your right shin toward your foot. As your left arm approaches being horizontal, feel a huge stretch along your whole left side. For an extra stretch, try to place your left palm on the back of your right hand. Now do the other side.

## Good Dog (Arfasana)

Roll over! Play dead! Sit! Beg! Lie down! Stay!

## Warped Plank (Distortasana)

There are at least five ways to avoid being flat from heels to head and thus to do this klutzier and asymmetrical version of chaturanga. Try to do them involuntarily, i.e., try to do a good plank, but fail. Bend like a bow, curve crookedly sideways, cramp into a kink, degenerate your thorax into a cup, or rubberize your spine into an uncontrolled twist.

## Swaybacked Nag (Rosinantasana)

This is just like the bow version of warped plank, except with a much deeper bend. Whinny as you inhale and trill an extended bilabial fricative as you exhale.

## Swinging Gate (Hinjasana)

From parighasana, lift your straight leg off the floor, keep it straight, let its arm slide down further toward your foot, and keep your other arm as near horizontal as possible. Now your only points of contact with the floor are the knee and instep of your bent leg. Balancing on these two contacts, swing your stiffened body back and forth, smoothly, without creaking. WD-40® might help.

## Locust (Salabhasana)

Lie comfortably in a prone position with your legs together and your arms by your sides. Tense your arms and either make fists or clasp your hands tightly together under your crotch. Tip your head back and try to touch the floor with your larynx. Your whole body should be centered and in line.

Inhale and slowly raise both legs together off the floor uniformly from your waist to your toes. Keep your legs absolutely straight. Above all, don't bend your knees. Exhale and lower your legs. Repeat.

As a variant, you could push your hands, either as fists or with palms flat down, into the floor by your sides, rather than under your crotch.

## Prone Boat (Naukasana)

From salabhasana, lift your arms straight out in front of you like a bowsprit. Find your drishti. Lift your chest like a prow. Your head is now a gallant figurehead. Set your course. Full speed ahead. Sweep your arms back like oars. Lift your legs higher and swab the poop deck. Balance on your navel.

You may wish to name this good ship the "S.S. Extreme Locust."

## Cockroach (Disgustasana)

From makarasana (page 42 above), while keeping your limbs all in the same horizontal plane with your body and keeping everything possible in contact with the floor, make cactus arms (page 16 above), bend your knees sharply, and bring them up to touch your elbows. Wiggle your fingers, toes, hands, feet, forearms, lower legs, eyebrows, tongue, etc., and randomly move all these parts, especially your elbows and knees, back and forth, up and down, in and out. Scuttle and scurry all around the room, skulking in corners and nooks.

This asana is a flat, floor-bound version of the mosquito (page 41 above). So, be as annoying as you wish.

Continue until crushed by a giant boot. Then go into a very flat savasana (page 74 below).

## Hovercraft (Aeronaukasana)

From naukasana, exhale and lift your belly up. Try to do this without lowering your legs, arms, chest, or head. In other words, try to achieve perfect horizontality by raising your middle rather than by lowering your extremities. You will fail - at least at first. Keep trying.

## Happy Baby (Ananda Balasana)

Lie on your back. Relax. Inhale. Stick all four limbs up in the air. Exhale. Hug your knees deep into your chest. Inhale. Grab and hook each big toe with the first two fingers of each hand. (This is the famous yoga toe lock, which is useful in so many asanas.) Keep your arms inside your legs. Exhale. Spread those thighs apart. Rock and roll. Back and forth. Round and round. Side to side. Ahhhhhh! Babble. Coo. Burble. Goo goo da da ma ma.

This asana is a wonderful massage for your back. All you need now is your blanky, your teddy, and your binky.

## Eye of the Needle (Sucirandhrasana)

From ananda balasana, let go of your toes and hug your knees to your chest. Put the outside of your right ankle on your left thigh just above the knee so that (from your point of view) your legs form an inverted figure four (4). Reach around your left leg with both arms - see why this asana is called "eye of the needle"? - and grab your left shin tight. Pull it in toward your chest as hard as you can. Feel that big stretch in your right hip.

Now do it on the other side.

## Colicky Baby (Screechi Belli Distendi Balasana)

This asana is the dangerous result of overusing the root lock (page 10 above) to the extent that doing the root unlock (page 11 above) becomes nearly impossible. Alas! Little can be done to comfort you if you reach this state. However, writhing in pain seems to produce some effect. Performing widely different asanas in rapid succession not only helps you to writhe, but is also the act of writhing itself.

From balasana (page 14 above), flip irrationally into dhanurasana (see next page). Don't forget to scream.

From dhanurasana, contort spasmodically into setubandhasana (page 22 above) and do the ups and downs without breathing properly.

From setubandhasana, roll over dizzyingly into bhujangasana (page 42 above), then bend agonizingly up into salabhasana, then awkwardly into naukasana (page 46 above).

From naukasana, give the perfect simhasana grimace (page 38 above), but try not to barf.

## Diaper Pin (Fibulasana)

Make sure your dhoti is well secured, or you will only increase your pain, both physically and psychologically. Bend over double and grab it.

## Bow (Dhanurasana)

Lie on your stomach with your knees only a little bit apart. Exhale. Bend your knees. Inhale. Reach back with both arms over your shoulders and grab your ankles. Exhale. Bend your chest and both legs up as high as they will go. Pull your soles toward the back of your head as close as they will come. Balance on your lower abdomen. Rock back and forth on your belly from your sternum to your pubic area. The pressure on your belly will not allow you to breathe normally, but don't worry about that. Just keep your breath steady and regular. Inhale on the backward rock and exhale on the forward rock, or vice versa, whichever suits you. Just make sure to coordinate your breathing somehow with your rocking.

Exhale, let go of your ankles, and return to an easy prone position.

## Shooting Bow (Akarna Dhanurasana)

From dandasana (page 22 above), lean forward and grab each big toe in the yoga toe lock. Keep one leg and its arm sticking out straight ahead, but pull your other leg every which way. Drag your foot back to your ear; haul it up over your head; shove it out to the side. Try - but fail - to dislocate your hip.

## Rifle (Remingtonasana)

Be perfectly still and steady, like a solidified tunnel (page 23 above). But if you merely solidify your tunnel, you will be a big bore. Try adjusting your caliber to become a small bore.

## Shooting Rifle (Akarna Ammo Remingtonasana)

There are four distinct asanas included under this name: prone, sitting, kneeling, and standing:

1. From sphinx (page 42 above), arrange your elbows on the floor so that you can comfortably bring your right thumb loosely to your right cheek, extend your left arm at about a 45-degree angle, and loosely form a cradle with your left palm.
2. In sukhasana (page 34 above), put your elbows on your knees, your right thumb loosely on your right cheek, and loosely form a left palm cradle.
3. Sit on your right heel. Put the left foot 90 degrees to the right leg so that the left shin is vertical. Rest the left elbow just beyond the left knee. Do the usual right thumb cheek and left palm cradle things.
4. From tadasana, do a right sidebend with a little backbend. Center yourself. Bring your right thumb loosely to your right cheek and lay your left elbow on your left side with its forearm vertical and its palm loosely forming a cradle.

Don't jerk your trigger; squeeeeeeeeze it.

## Half Moon (Ardha Chandrasana)

This asana is the ultimate sidebend. From urdhva hastasana (page 12 above), exhale, push your left hip outward while pushing everything from the waist up over to the right as far as you can while keeping your hands together, your arms straight, and your body all in one plane. That is, don't bend either forward or backward. If you've done it right, you should resemble a waxing crescent moon.

Inhale and return to urdhva hastasana. Exhale and bend to the other side, so that you now resemble a waning crescent moon. Repeat the cycle. Da capo.

## Revolving Half Moon (Parivrtta Ardha Chandrasana)

From parivrtta trikonasana (page 28 above), instead of keeping both feet on the floor and turning to one side or the other, balance on one foot, bend sharply sideways from the waist so that your arms are in line and vertical, one hand on the floor and the other reaching for the sky, and so that your torso and your other leg are in line. Now do it on the other side.

You can also go into this asana from virabhadrasana III (page 72 below). After all, it looks sort of like a sideways warrior III.

## Full Moon (Puffasana)

Inhale as deeply and as long as you possibly can, filling with air first the belly, then the lower lungs, then the middle lungs, then the upper lungs, then the mouth, pharynx, eustachian tubes, and so on, until all your bodily channels are engorged and your skin separates from your body like that of a Peking duck. You should now be perfectly spherical. Be serene as you contemplate your new spatiality and the ultimate unity and plenitude that it represents.

## New Moon (Flabbiflappasana)

From full moon, exhale completely in a gigantic WHOOSH! - like suddenly letting the air out of an untied balloon. You involuntarily and haphazardly flit around the room. Enjoy your flight!

Again, be serene as you contemplate the essential emptiness and nothingness of the universe, now represented by your airless body. If you're lucky, your skin may reattach.

## Plumber's Moon (Hafmastassasana)

Do upavesasana (page 56 below), but make sure that the drawstring on your yoga pants is loose. Better still, wear low-slung ragged jeans without a belt.

### Chair (Utkatasana)

From any standing position, preferably tadasana, press your legs together and, with a mighty inhale, swing both arms in unison up in front of you and over your head. Exhale and squat down with your chest as high as possible, and with your torso and thighs at a 90-degree angle, ideally with the thighs horizontal and the torso vertical. Tense up! But keep breathing! Your body, from a side view, should now resemble a chair without its two back legs.

Hold still as long as possible. If this doesn't firm up your quads, nothing will.

### Table (Bharmanasana)

As promised on page 18 above, here is the basic asana in-between cat and cow. It's really not much more complicated than getting down on your hands and knees, but you must remember to breathe.

### Balancing Table (Dandayamna Bharmanasana)

From bharmanasana, inhale and stick your right leg and left arm straight out horizontally. Hold this pose for a few breaths, then exhale and bring them back down. Inhale and do it with the opposite limbs. Hold it, exhale, and bring them down. Repeat.

## Couch (Potatasana)

Lie on your right side with your upper right arm in line with your body and resting on the floor, your right elbow bent, and the right side of your head resting on your right palm. Hold this pose as long as you like. Have plenty of your favorite snacks and beverages, just the way you like them, within easy reach of your left hand. The key word - the mantra - for this asana is "comfort." Whenever you feel the least bit of discomfort, flip over and do all this on your left side. Have lots of pillows handy if you need them.

Your drishti is black, flat, and rectangular, with an 80-inch diagonal. You are in the perfect position to see it all clearly.

## Coffee Table (Longbharmanasana)

This asana is like bharmanasana, except that you get down lower. There are several ways to achieve this lowering while still keeping a horizontal back; however, none are reliable and many cause serious injury. Just do your best and try to look decorative.

When there are five of you, four could be chairs around the fifth, the table. Don't forget to bring a deck of cards.

## Garland Squat (Upavesasana or Maalaasana)

Stand comfortably with your legs about twice hip distance apart and your feet at 45-degree angles. Squat down as low as you can without your butt touching the floor. Bring your hands together at your heart center, in either traditional prayer position or uttarabodhi (page 60 below). Your elbows should be sticking straight out, resting either on your knees or just in front of them. Keep your feet flat on the floor.

If you want, you can exhale, lean forward without losing your balance, wrap your arms around the outside of your knees, reach around, clasp your hands behind your lower back, inhale, and lift your head and chest up. Good luck!

The word "upavesa" means "sitting," so this is the "sitting pose." The word "maalaa" (note the doubled vowels) means "garland," so this is the "garland pose," because the arms hang down in front like a garland. But this squat is also called "malasana" (with no doubled vowels), which literally means "shitting pose." No shit! In Sanskrit, the noun "mala" means "dirt, excrement, bad stuff," just as the Latin prefix "mal-" means "bad" and the Greek adjective "kakos" means "bad, evil, vile, vulgar, nasty." Why do you think little kids call their poop "caca" in French, Spanish, and English; "cacca" in Italian; and "Kacke" in German? And why is it called "malodorous"?

## Pete Rose (Battabattabattasana)

From utkatasana (page 54 above), squat down even lower and deeper, but not as low or as deep as upavesasana. Keep your legs energized and engaged. Make two fists in front of you. Put the bottom of your right fist on the top of your left fist, as if grasping a baseball bat. Keep your fists together as you bring them behind your right ear. Feel the stretch in your left shoulder. Gaze sideways over your left shoulder and scowl menacingly but confidently. Be tense and relaxed at the same time. Be a bit cocky. Actually, be very cocky.

Swing!

Get back into your low, deep squat with your legs still energized and engaged. Again make the two fists, but this time put the left on top of the right. (Pete was a switch hitter.) Bring them behind your left ear. Feel the stretch in your right shoulder. Gaze sideways over your right shoulder with the same menacing, confident scowl. Remember to stay both tense and relaxed. Be really really cocky - even to the point of giving cockiness a new definition.

Swing!

Repeat until you get 4256 hits.

## Crane (Bakasana) or Crow (Kakasana)

From upavesasana (page 56 above), either put your armpits inside your knees or your knees outside your armpits, depending on how you look at it. Put your palms on the floor directly beneath your shoulders with your hands pointing forward. Spread your fingers as wide as possible. With your weight on your wrists, begin to tip forward, slowly, deliberately, and always under control.

Find your drishti. Lift your butt up. Balance on your wrists and tiptoes. Keep your head up and centered. Breathe.

For bakasana, your upper shins should now be on the backs of your upper arms, as close to the armpits as possible. For kakasana, your knees should now be in your armpits.

Keep tipping forward, with your focus steady on your drishti, until your toes leave the floor. Balance on your wrists. Breathe normally for as long as you can hold this pose, then exhale slowly as you lower yourself back down into upavesasana.

Bakasana or kakasana builds upper body strength, especially in the forearms. It also enhances concentration and improves circulation.

## Turkey (Klutzasana)

From bakasana or kakasana, walk around on your hands. Fall on your face. Shake your wattle. Squat and gobble.

## Gull (Stukasana)

Spread your wings. Inhale. Take off! Glide! Swoop! Soar! Dive! Be the essence of grace.

## Albatross (Gooniasana)

This is a cross between turkey and gull, i.e., a really klutzy gull, the antithesis of grace. But don't feel bad about it. Spread your wings anyway. Inhale. Stretch 'em out. Way out. Get big. Try to take off. Fall on your face.

Try it again. Be resolute! Focus! Succeed! Glide! Swoop! Soar! Dive! Now you're even more the essence of grace than the gull.

## Hummingbird (Nektasukkasana)

Get small. Flap your wings real fast. Hyperventilate. Be in two places at once. Be beautiful, delicate, and iridescent, but not at all annoying like the mosquito (page 41 above).

## Mudras

Mudras are yoga for your hands. Various shapes of the hands align with the chakras and energy paths to promote serenity and health. A few examples:

### Enlightenment Mudra (Uttarabodhi)

Clasp your hands with the fingers interlaced, except that the two index fingers are together, pointing up like a steeple, and your two thumbs are together, in line with your index fingers, and pointing down, 180 degrees away from them. Lay the sides of your index fingers and thumbs directly over your heart center. This mudra can be used instead of the usual prayer hands if you prefer reason to faith.

### Unity Seal (Yoga Mudra)

The yoga mudra is the symbol of yoga. From either virasana (page 16 above), or padmasana (page 34 above), clasp your hands behind your back with your thumbs sticking straight out together and lying along the crack of your butt. Inhale. Keep your arms straight. Focus on your third eye. Exhale. Bend forward from the waist as far as you can, ideally so that your third eye touches the floor. Your arms should now be vertical and your thumbs horizontal. In the late Middle Ages, this was called strappado.

## Bronx Mudra (Razberi)

With your hand perpendicular to your face, inhale, spread your four fingers wide, stick them upward, and hook the tip of your upturned thumb under the tip of your nose. With a huge, loud exhale, put your tongue between your protruding lips, make the rude noise commonly known as a raspberry, and wiggle your fingers mockingly back and forth.

## Nanker Mudra (Phelji)

Put one hand in front of your face with your chin in your palm and and your thumb and pinky stretched out along the line of your jaw. With your middle finger, push the tip of your nose skyward so that anyone looking at you can see up your nostrils all the way to your pharynx. With your index and ring fingers, pull your cheek skin down on both sides so that your eyeballs seem gigantic, thus preventing anyone from wanting to look at you. This mudra was devised by Brian Jones (1942-1969), founder of the Rolling Stones. Strewth!

## Wanker Mudra (Mastabati)

For a description of this mudra, you'll have to wait until the unexpurgated version of this book appears. Meanwhile, use your imagination. Being British helps.

## Camel (Ustrasana)

From virasana (page 16 above), inhale and rise up so that you are sort of standing on your knees. Put your hands on your hips, arms akimbo, inhale, and do a little backbend. Reach, first up, then behind, with both hands and grab your heels. Pull your body back as far as you can. Expand your ribs, push your heels down, toss your head back, pull your spine down toward your calves, squish your butt cheeks together, and stretch your neck out, all as far as you can. Gaze at the ceiling or the sky, as the case may be. Try to make your torso horizontal while keeping your thighs vertical.

This is an excellent stretch for the spine, hips, and shoulders. It is also a pretty good way to cause yourself intense discomfort, However, as with all asanas, stop short of creating great pain. Yes, we know, "No pain, no gain!" But asanas are not body-building calisthenics. They are a means to breathe.

Why this asana is called the "camel" is a mystery. Who has ever seen a real camel in this position? Camels typically just schlep around, mocking the desert, spitting, sneering, biting, making lots of noise, being bad-tempered, and having, if they are bactrians, two humps, or if they are dromedaries, one hump. Where is there a hump in this asana?

## Realistic Camel I (Dromedariasana)

To develop incredible spinal flexibility, let's try the following three variants of the cat-cow asana pair (page 18 above).

Whereas in cat, your head is down and your spine is up, and whereas in cow, your head is up and your spine is down, you can make a realistic camel by putting your head and spine up both at the same time. But then you must also act like a camel. They have very bad tempers. So will you in this position.

Fervent astrologers may wish to perform this asana on Wednesday, which is hump day.

Whatever you do, don't get stuck in this pose! That would be the dreaded involuntary hunchback pose (quasimodoasana), to be avoided at all costs.

## Realistic Camel II (Bactrianasana)

Same as above, but with two humps in your spine.

## Loch Ness Monster (Undulatasana)

Same as above, but with three or more humps in your spine. This requires supreme control. Do it, be cool, and you will truly surpass yourself.

## Pigeon (Kapotasana)

From virasana (page 16 above), puff out your chest like a proud strutting pigeon. Bend backwards, grab your feet, breathe, and pull yourself back.

But, you may ask, isn't this like the camel (page 62 above)? Almost, but not quite. The pigeon gives a deeper backbend. In ustrasana, the arms finish straight, vertical, and with the palms on the heels; but in kapotasana, the arms finish bent, with the elbows on the floor and the hands grabbing either the heels or the ankles.

## One-Legged King Pigeon (Eka Pada Rajakapotasana)

From downward dog (page 40 above), inhale the right knee between your arms, bringing your right heel as close to your crotch as possible, then exhale both legs slowly down, so that the outside of the right leg and the top of the left leg rest on the floor. Sit tall. Bend your left knee so that your left calf is vertical. Exhale. Reach back over your head, grab your left ankle with both hands, and pull your torso back. Be sure to keep your hips square and forward throughout this whole process. Release your ankle, relax, go back into downward dog, then be the one-legged king pigeon on the other side.

## Stool Pigeon (Informasana)

From coward (page 17 above), emerge into utkatasana (page 54 above). Sing. Slump back down into coward. Repeat.

## Cement-Shoes Stool Pigeon (Exinformasana)

There are two ways to do this asana, either in reality or in your imagination. Since doing it in reality is always fatal, we recommend doing it only in your imagination.

Stand in tadasana. You are in New York City at the end of an East River pier in the wee small hours of a moonless night, surrounded by three burly, scowling goons who look like extras from a B mobster movie. Two of them stand on either side of you so that you can't move or make any noise, while the third mixes quick-set cement in a bucket. Stay firm in tadasana. Don't whine. Don't sob. Above all, don't dissolve into coward. Be a shining example for all stool pigeons.

The two on each side pick you straight up under the armpits and put your feet in the bucket. The cement sets. Stay in tadasana. They pick you straight up and drop you in the river. Try to enjoy watching the fish. You can't. It's dark. Try to breathe. You can't. Expire gracefully. Don't go back into coward.

## Frog (Bhekasana)

Bhekasana is a very difficult quadriceps stretch. To ease into it, first perform virasana, dhanurasana, ustrasana, ananda balasana, natarajasana, utthita hasta padangusthasana, setubandhasana, navasana, upavesasana, garudasana, salabhasana, utkatasana, alanasana, and anything else you want, in any order you want. Anything to loosen it all up!

Once prepared, lie prone with your feet about hip width apart and your arms by your sides, palms down. Exhale, bend your knees sharply, trying to touch your buttocks with your heels. Put your palms on top of your insteps. Now turn your wrists 180 degrees so that your toes and fingers are all pointing toward your shoulders and your palms are on top of your toes. Push down hard! Try to push your soles into the floor. Try to break your feet. Do a backbend and raise your chest and head.

You should now look like a sitting frog and feel like a gigged frog. Keep pushing. Keep breathing. Keep stretching your quads, balancing on your belly, squashing your manipura and svadhishthana, and ruining your knees. Smile! Remain in this position for five or ten minutes, which will seem like as many hours. Don't croak! Exhale yourself out of this torment and relax. You've earned it.

## Frogs (Brekekekexkoaxkoaxasana)

In navasana (page 32 above) or naukasana (page 46 above), imagine that you are a boat crossing the mythic River Styx in the underworld. The oarsman, Charon (pronounced "Karen"), looks quite annoyed. Having done this ferrying for millennia already, he is sick and tired of hearing what the Stygian frogs consider their sacred sound. It's not "Om"; it's more like the sacred sound of the root unlock.

Fascinated, mesmerized, you and all your fellow yogis morph into these frogs. Your jaws gape open. Your sense of the sarcastic becomes more acute. You sing hideous burbling, gurgling noises which seem to you as beautiful as the sweetest hymn.
Brekekekex koax koax!
You croak but you do not croak.
Brekekekex koax koax!
You hop around on all fours. You splash and dive in the rancid waters.
Brekekekex koax koax!
You continue to sing.
Brekekekex koax koax!
Your sacred sound becomes deafening.
Brekekekex koax koax!
You morph back into navasana, which has now reached the far shore. Charon demands his fare.
Pay up!

## Warrior I (Virabhadrasana I)

From tadasana, take a giant step - almost a leap - back with your right leg, bringing it just slightly outward, keeping it straight, but turning your right foot to about a 45-degree angle. Keep your hips, left foot, torso, and head all facing forward. Your left shin should be vertical, your left thigh horizontal, and your left knee at a 90-degree angle. Once again recall the invisible string pulling you up through the crown of your head. You must be able to see the tips of your left toes beyond your left knee without tilting your face forward or pulling your knee back.

With your back foot firmly grounded, inhale your arms straight up over your head, palms facing each other about shoulder width apart. Keep your chest high and your gaze forward, but maybe add a little backbend and a little backward tilt of your head, looking at your hands. Exhale, straighten your left leg, and swing your arms loosely down to your sides, keeping your shoulders soft. Repeat. This is called "warrior flow." Throughout this entire process, be sure that your spine stays long, your butt is tucked down, your shoulders are rolled back and down, and your weight is on your back leg. When you're done with the flow, exhale and leap back into tadasana.

Now do the whole thing on the other side.

## Wounded Warrior I (Kiasana)

From virabhadrasana I, suddenly clutch any vital part of your body and yell, "They got me!" as loud as your rapidly fading powers allow. Fall down willy-nilly, continue your agonized and agonizing screams, writhe every which way like a colicky baby (page 49 above), and add any other supine, near-supine, prone, near-prone, sideways, twisted, bent, inverted, perverted, shameless, or ground-hugging contortions you wish. Get used to it, because you will soon be hugging the ground from six feet under.

Mustering as much self-pity as possible, eulogize yourself:

"Thou art the ruins of the noblest man
That ever lived in the tide of times.
Woe to the hand that shed this costly blood! ...
A curse shall light upon the limbs of men;
Domestic fury and fierce civil strife ...
Blood and destruction shall be so in use
And dreadful objects so familiar
That mothers shall but smile when they behold
Their infants quarter'd with the hands of war ...
That this foul deed shall smell above the earth
With carrion men, groaning for burial."

- Shakespeare, *Julius Caesar*, III, i, 256-275

Go into savasana (page 74 below).

## Warrior II (Virabhadrasana II)

This is almost like warrior I, except that the body is turned mostly toward the side instead of toward the front; so, from tadasana, take that leap back with your right leg, but turn your right foot to about a 90-degree angle and turn your hips to the side.

Inhale both arms straight out horizontally, palms down, extending them as far as possible, in the same plane as your body. Turn your head forward. Gaze over your front shoulder, elbow, and middle finger, which should be all in line. Pull your head back slightly, but always remember the invisible string.

## Rag Doll (Ardha Uttanasana)

From tadasana (page 12 above), soften your knees a bit, grab opposite elbows in front of you, exhale slowly, hang your head down, and bend forward as far as you can, but gently, without forcing anything. Let everything above your waist just dangle, limp, loose, letting gravity do all the work.

Inhale slowly and roll it all back up into tadasana, one vertebra at a time.

This is a great exercise to stretch the spine and hamstrings and improve their flexibility.

## Wounded Warrior II (Amputatasana)

From virabhadrasana II, without moving any other part of your body, bend the knee of your back (right) leg so that its heel touches your right butt cheek. Breathe, Balance. Stay calm. Hold that pose. Focus on your drishti. Remember that string.

If all this seems physically impossible, and even if you fall down a thousand times while trying it, be persistent. As you persist, meditate on the fact that real amputees can do seemingly impossible things.

If you don't believe it, go watch a wheelchair basketball game. Be amazed.

## Barbie® Doll (Bimboasana)

If you are a woman, suck in some parts, puff out other parts, develop parts that don't exist, pretend that non-existent parts actually do exist, and do your best to look unrealistic.

## Ken® Doll (Sissiasana)

If you are a man, forget that you are. Inhale your genitalia up into your abdomen. Try to look as phony, simpering, and unmanly as possible, as if you never had an original thought in your life.

## Warrior III (Virabhadrasana III)

From virabhadrasana I (page 68 above), inhale and straighten your bent leg so that it now serves as your front leg. With your arms still extended over your head and just next to your ears, exhale, bend slowly forward, and lift your back leg off the floor so that everything from your fingertips to the heel of your back foot is in line. Inhale and stabilize. Exhale and keep bending forward until your front leg is vertical, everything else is horizontal, and you are naturally looking down. Your body, seen from the side, should now resemble a capital "T."

Alternately, from urdhva hastasana (page 12 above), exhale while bending slightly forward, keeping one leg vertical and firmly rooted to the floor, but allowing the other to rise. Inhale, stabilize, exhale, bend forward, establish alignment, and come into that capital "T."

Once you have achieved warrior III, you will have many options for further movement and flow. For example, bring both arms back 135 degrees, but keep them horizontal, ending up with "airplane arms" at 45-degree angles to your body, like a delta-winged fighter jet. From that asana you can sweep up into utkatasana (page 54 above). Then you can repeat the whole process with the other foot on the floor.

## Wounded Warrior III (Belliflopppasana)

From virabhadrasana III, kick your standing leg out behind you and fall - Splat!

Or perhaps you would rather absorb what the *Hitchhiker's Guide to the Galaxy* has to say on the subject: "The knack lies in learning how to throw yourself at the ground and miss. ... All it requires is simply the ability to throw yourself forward with all your weight, and the willingness not to mind that it's going to hurt. ... Most people fall to miss the ground, and if they are really trying properly, the likelihood is that they will fail to miss it fairly hard. ... One problem is that you have to miss the ground accidentally. It's no good deliberately intending to miss the ground because you won't. You have to have your attention suddenly distracted by something else when you're halfway there, so that you are no longer thinking about falling, or about the ground, or about how much it's going to hurt if you fail to miss it. It is notoriously difficult to prize your attention away from these three things during the split second you have at your disposal. ... Ignore all considerations of your own weight and simply let yourself waft higher. ... Waft higher and higher ... then drift above the treetops breathing regularly."

- Douglas Adams, *Life, the Universe, and Everything* (New York: Ballantine, 1982), pp. 75-77

## Corpse (Savasana)

Some say that all asanas are a preparation for savasana. Well, maybe that's true of the wounded warriors and the dying Gaul - but, in any case, savasana is a cool pose. You don't even do anything! You just lie there on your back. Breathing. Chilling. Relaxing. Falling asleep. But not dying. Not really.

Lie supine with your legs and arms straight, soft, and comfortably apart. Take a long, slow, colossal inhale and tighten everything up. Then with one big, fat, giant, loud exhale - **WHOOSH!** - let it all go. Melt into the floor. Softly close your eyes. Listen to your breath. Let your legs rest comfortably apart. Let your feet fall outward. Let your hands fall loosely open, palms up. Roll your head gently from side to side until it finds its place. Don't be surprised if you feel so relaxed that you fall asleep.

You may want to enhance your relaxation even more. If so, then try any of these before you take that Brobdingnagian inhale: Put an eyeshade over your face. Put a pillow under your knees to flatten and lengthen your spine. Put a drop of essential oil on your third eye for aromatherapy. Put pads under the backs of your hands. Put a cool compress on your forehead. Or cover yourself with a blanket - not a shroud - a blanket. You're not a real corpse yet.

## Reverse Hovercraft (Aeronavasana)

If you've accomplished savasana correctly, you should now be so relaxed that anything is possible. You are completely in touch with yourself, with the earth, with the whole universe. Keep breathing. That's the key. Slowly, slowly inhale; slowly, slowly exhale, then do it again, slowly, slowly, slowly. Stay in focus without focus. Do by not doing. Act by not acting, Breathe without breathing. Think without thinking. Be without being.

Throw yourself at the sky and don't miss.

Any multi-occurring phenomenon that we either experience or perform, if we wish to honor it, we call consistent, reliable, or productive of desired results; but if we speak pejoratively of it or wish to disparage it, we call it repetitive, tedious, or say that it produces nothing but ennui. We all strive to be consistent and to perform reliably, but when we fail, we may sometimes take a "sour grapes" view of our failure: "Oh well, that was boring anyway."

So it may be with yoga.

But this book isn't called *Yoga for Fools* for no reason. To wallow in failure, or to shrug it off, is the essence of foolishness.

**Namaste!**